His Foods

My Journey Back to Health

Norma Jean

Dedicated to you... my reader.

May the pages of this book give you hope.

Hope you can lose weight when you have given up. Hope for a life with less pain, whether in your body or in your heart, and a belief in the healing power of the body.

Disclaimer

This book is meant only to share my personal experiences and to introduce you to some of the resources I have relied upon over the years. There are many other resources available to you; and I urge you to continue to explore them in order to find answers to your own personal issues when dealing with food and food combining.

<u>Any information disseminated is meant to dispense knowledge only. If you need medical attention, please consult your doctor or other health care professional.</u>

Any discussion of food combinations and choices should include the reality that a great deal of criticism has been leveled at the safety and quality of the food supply. The food industry would argue that the criticism is an exaggeration based on assumptions and anecdotal evidence. Anyone familiar with the food supply would have to agree that today's products are not the same as those from forty years ago. The need for an increased food supply to keep up with the growth of the world's population has led to significant advancements and changes in the use of genetic and chemical processes.

My advice to you continues to be: "Listen to your body." If a food item bothers you, your body will tell you so. Also as a part of your decision-making process, I would encourage you to include your doctor in the discussion.

Acknowledgements

When I moved to Florida, I met wonderful new neighbors who welcomed me, learned that I had a passion for helping people lead healthier and happier lives, had success with my program, and encouraged me to put my story in print, which had been only a dream of mine up to that point.

Gerry and Meryle, thank you for believing in my message and for the hours and months of help that brought it to print. You encouraged and supported me throughout the year of writing. You both mean so much to me.

Thank you to Sandy, Carmelita, and Sally who time and time again were there whenever I needed someone to re-read a chapter and offer suggestions. Your rewrites in those early days made me a more focused writer. George and Gloria, thank you for all your help. I had a dream to share and you found a way to translate that dream into the pages of this book.

I will always be grateful to the staff at The Lifelong Learning College in The Villages, Florida. Thank you also to my many students who kept me focused on a path of continuing to help others. It is my hope that many of you will have the same success I have had with this program, and you continue to share those successes with me.

A very special thank you to my husband Howard, whose support never waivered throughout the year of writing, and to my daughter Rachael; who worked tirelessly on formatting. Your visit was no coincidence. You came at a time when I needed your help the most.

And most importantly I thank GOD. I had so many questions and doubts over the years; but there was always a plan and you directed me toward those who could help me achieve that plan. I owe my health to your whole foods and your design of the body. One recent day in church, my roaming mind was suddenly brought back to the words spoken from the altar.

"By the river on its bank, on one side and on the other, will grow all kinds of trees for food. Their leaves will not wither and their fruit will not fail. They will bear every month because their water flows from the sanctuary and their fruit will be for food and their leaves for healing."

Ezekiel 47:12

Thank you for blessing me with a journey to share with others.

CONTENTS

Introduction

Whenever I eat a food, plan a meal at home, or dine out, I have two thoughts in mind: What foods are correct for my blood type, (type A), and how to combine those foods to digest well. These are the two most important choices I make each day. If meals do not digest properly, toxins are created in the body; and over time, this can hinder the body's natural healing process and lead to numerous health problems.

I retired a few years ago, having enjoyed excellent health for quite some time; but it was not always that way. This book will explain the program I have followed for many years and will provide a guide for you to use whether dining at home or in a restaurant. Meals for each blood type, properly combined for optimum digestion, are included.

Today it has become common to eat a "Thanksgiving type meal" as many as three times a day, further taxing an already overburdened and aging system. The meal combines many types of foods: carbohydrates (bread, rice, potatoes), fats (oil or butter), and proteins, (eggs, beef, chicken, fish).

When these foods are combined improperly, the results are uncomfortable symptoms we are all too familiar with. On the other hand, when digestion occurs easily with proper food combining, there is no bloating, indigestion, or fatigue.

Each of our systems may be at a different stage of health or disease within the body; and we may not even know there is an issue until a problem is found by the doctor. However, one thing is certain. The digestive system and the body sent warning signs, time and time again, which were not recognized or were ignored. I indicated earlier that I was not always in optimum health. I had many of the same problems you might be experiencing. When I learned what was causing uncomfortable feelings after eating and corrected my diet, many things changed. The bloating, asthma, and allergy symptoms I had for years disappeared, and so did the extra weight. More importantly, the muscle and joint pain I experienced was gone.

Whole foods never come with ingredient labels. They have no side effects unless a food is wrong for a blood type, or is incorrectly combined with other foods. As I shared a meal with friends recently at a local restaurant, I ordered foods correct for my blood type and I properly combined foods to aid digestion. I had no discomfort during or after the meal. I wondered if my friends felt the same after they returned home.

Retirement is sometimes sobering. Moments of joy can change to times of great concern if our health begins to fail. As we age, so do the organs of digestion. We are reminded of this fact, after a meal. Sales of digestive aids in recent years have skyrocketed, becoming the largest over the counter medications sold. Taking a moment to think about foods, or the meal we are about to eat, becomes more important as we age. Our choices will either hinder or aid digestion and ultimately affect our overall health.

This book is not about giving up any food or drink. It is about understanding how to enjoy them so we don't compromise the body's ability to keep us healthy. It's not what we do 20% of the time that hurts us; it's what we do the other 80% that does.

I make correct choices because long ago I experienced the results of not doing that. I don't want the pain or uncomfortable symptoms to return. Last but not least, I certainly do not want to regain the weight I lost. When someone pays me a compliment about looking younger than I am, my reply is "It's *all* about food".

Chapter One
My Journey Begins

NORMA JEAN

Norma Jean,

"...I had my yearly physical today, and like you, all my numbers were improved over the results from one year ago. Every category...was rated desirable or best. I told him (the doctor) it was the knowledge imparted through your class at The (Lifelong) Learning College ..."

Carol B.
The Villages, FL.

Eating meals containing foods right for my blood type became a way of life many years ago. It was in a gym where many of us shared information about diet and health, when I first heard about "Eat Right 4 Your Type" by Dr. Peter J. D'Adamo. The book explains the link our genetic heritage has to diet, and how different foods affect each individual blood type. From Dr. D'Adamo, "Each blood type contains the genetic message of our ancestors' diets and behaviors, and though we're a long way away from early history, many of their traits still affect us".

A friend with Type B blood once mentioned she never quite felt right after eating chicken. Chicken contains a protein, or lectin in its muscle tissue which affects those with this blood type. Eating chicken is not a good idea for those with blood type B, as the lectin attacks the bloodstream and can lead to immune disorders. Turkey does not contain this lectin and is a much healthier choice.

Another example of an "avoid" food for a particular blood type is wheat. Gluten-free foods are everywhere today. The *protein*, or *lectin* found in wheat, barley and rye is *gluten*. It contains a specific type of lectin and has been linked to rheumatoid arthritis. Though other blood types can be sensitive to gluten, it can be especially troublesome for those with blood type O, or for anyone with celiac disease. These are two examples of how different blood types react to foods that should be at best eliminated or at least reduced.

As the doctor states in his book, lectins can be a dangerous "*glue*" leading to a host of health problems. These "sticky" molecules bind to tissues in the body or the intestine. The condition known as leaky gut syndrome occurs when the intestinal lining becomes damaged from these foreign invaders. A small percentage of lectins also circulate into the bloodstream causing food allergies, inflammation and even weight gain.

I never knew the gentleman's name in the gym that day. I hope I thanked him, for he was right. It did not take long for me to realize what one person can eat, another cannot. This was the beginning of a program which would impact my health in many ways. I had been eating the wrong foods for my blood type and it all came down to the wrong protein.

When we think of protein, what comes to mind is chicken, beef, fish, eggs and dairy; but almost all foods contain protein in small amounts. For instance, there are 1.3 grams of protein in a banana and 2.1 grams of protein in a sweet potato; yet I rarely eat these foods because they are wrong for my blood type. The body targets these foreign particles as the blood begins to clump the cells together in an effort to eliminate them. In Dr. D'Adamo's words, "...when you eat a food containing protein lectins that are incompatible with your blood type antigen, the lectins target an organ or bodily system (kidneys, liver, brain, stomach, etc.) and begin to agglutinate blood cells in that area." I recommend Dr. D'Adamo's book for further understanding of the science and the explanation of this process which affects our health in many ways.

Some of the books I have read recently suggest limiting foods which cause digestive problems and allergic responses; and they refer to these foods as "incompatible foods" or to the problem as "food intolerance." To address these two issues these problematic foods are eliminated for a time and then slowly re-introduced. I found it easier to simply learn my "avoid" foods and eliminate *them*.

To keep this simple and easy for a healthy dining experience at home or in a restaurant, I have selected the correct foods for each blood type. The most important part is that the entire meal is properly combined for you. No matter what foods are chosen, these foods must digest to send the necessary nutrients for cellular health. Said another way, if I choose all the correct foods for my blood type and these foods do not digest well, toxins will be circulated into the body instead of nutrients. Our body uses a great deal of energy to digest a meal. It is a difficult process. This is one reason we feel fatigued after eating a meal of too many different types of foods. The body is having quite a time digesting the meal.

When I began eliminating most of my "avoid" foods, I saw immediate improvement in my health, especially my allergies. After being on steroids and prescription inhalers for years and enduring many seasonal coughs and colds, I have been free from asthma and allergies for a very long time and cannot remember the last time I had a cold. Do I ever eat some of these avoid foods for my type A blood? Of course I do, occasionally. I have found enjoying an *occasional* avoid food posses little harm. Eating them often does.

When it comes to decisions about whether to add an occasional avoid food into my diet, I consider whether the benefits are too numerous to ignore as in the case of unrefined coconut oil. Adding this oil promotes fat *loss*, provides energy and is chemically stable for use in cooking. This very beneficial oil is deserving of its own book and there are many. One I highly recommend is "The Coconut Oil Miracle," by Bruce Fife, N.D. He states, "When coconut oil is eaten, the body transforms its unique fatty acids into antimicrobial powerhouses capable of defeating some of the most notorious disease causing microorganisims...the unique properties of coconut oil make it, in essence, a natural antibacterial anti-fungal, and antiprotosoal food".

I use it on my skin and in my diet. It is listed as an avoid for type O blood. In some books it is even listed as an avoid for my own blood type A; yet in other books it is not. The decision I came to after much research was to include coconut oil in my diet, and I have for many years. If you still choose to avoid coconut oil after reading the above benefits, another healthy fat is ghee. Ghee, from grass fed cows, is clarified butter with the milk solids and impurities removed. It is rich in K2 for bone health, and CLA which is an antioxidant with anti viral properties. Ghee is rich in vitamin A, D, and E and is well tolerated by those with lactose or casein intolerance.

"NATURAL FORCES WITHIN US ARE THE TRUE
HEALERS OF DISEASE."

HIPPOCRATES

I had been eating right for my blood type A for many years before moving to California about the year 2000. I hadn't at that time studied natural health; however as an aesthetician for many years, I began attending conventions with dermatologists and plastic surgeons. This is when I realized the influence that diet has on the skin.

The skin is an organ, and I was beginning to look at it in a very different way. No longer was I only interested in treating the skin topically with procedures and products, I wanted to understand the skin from within. I soon realized the external damage seen as wrinkling and sagging not only happened from too much sun exposure, it also happened due to a process from within the body.

Make no mistake about the main cause of wrinkling and sagging skin. The sun is responsible for 80% of the aging of the skin due to inflammation from excess sun exposure. However, damage also occurs to the skin from glycation. Glycation is short for *A*dvanced *G*lycosylation *E*nd Product(s) and is a result of excess sugar circulating in the blood which causes collagen and elastin, the support structures of the skin to collapse and sag. Lo and behold we have wrinkles. Thus preventing this process through our diet leads to a more youthful appearance. It is so important, not only for the health of the skin, but for the entire body.

Over ten years ago I wrote two papers for aestheticians on this subject for <u>Dermascope</u> magazine. The most recent one published in November, 2007 is included in the Appendix.

It was during Dr. Nicholas Perricone's anti-aging conventions where I learned more about inflammation and the effect it has on the skin and body. I can remember him stating it would be years before mainstream media, as well as the medical establishment, would recognize the damaging effects of the inflammatory process on the body.

Twenty years after those first conventions I thought of Dr. Perricone. While watching nightly news one evening a doctor was interviewed about the link between smoking and other diseases. As disease after disease scrolled across the TV screen, he was asked about the connection. The link to lung cancer was well established but why all these other diseases? His answer contained a word I heard from the doctor many years earlier at those anti-aging conventions …*inflammation*...the root cause of so many of today's lifestyle diseases.

Inflammation is what happens when you sunburn. Some inflammatory processes are necessary and helpful. Our body heals a wound or cut with the process of inflammation; however, the danger to our health lies in chronic inflammation occurring on the cellular level deep within the body.

To this day, I can picture Dr. Perricone at that podium lecturing his peers about the common denominator in lifestyle diseases of heart, cancer, stroke, diabetes, and alzheimer's. It is inflammation. He was right, it took years to be recognized as a major contributor to poor health today.

A second member of my family was about to fight one of the above diseases. While I was in California I received a call from my brother saying he had been recently diagnosed with a rare cancer. I recall this conversation well. I can remember thinking I hadn't been able to do anything to help my mom who died at a very young age from cancer; but this time I was determined to learn all I could to help my brother.

From the conventions with the doctors, I had begun to understand how food affected not only the skin but the health of the body, so I realized food would hold the best chance for a return to health for my brother.

I had never heard of food combining until I headed to a local health store in California. I was discussing supplements for my brother with the store owner, when the conversation turned to diet. As we talked about nutrition, she guided me to an area of books about food combining. There were many books to choose from that day and I have read quite a few since then. There are even more charts about combinations of foods than there are books. The food combining tables within this book are what I have followed for many years to retain wonderful health. I follow them 80 to 90% of the time.

"I have followed food combining for years. Gone was 20 pounds...gone was bloating...gone was IBS."

Kathryn G.
The Villages, FL.

This is the concept behind food combining: if meals do not digest properly, the result is fermentation, leading to toxic undigested residue in the digestive tract. Undigested food can be seen as weight gain and cellulite and can be felt as bloating and indigestion as the body struggles to digest the food down to the most minute particle size for use in the cells. Uncomfortable symptoms from a poorly digested meal are most often caused by improper food combinations.

Imagine meal after meal where this is happening. When a meal is digesting correctly with proper food combinations, no symptoms are felt. No bloating, no gas, no indigestion, and no fatigue. Properly digested meals deliver nutrients that help the body heal. This is the most important reason to combine foods properly. I found the answer for my brother so I traveled to Pennsylvania to help him in his fight to regain health. This is what I was looking for when I was in the health store that day in California.

While the doctors did what they could, we did the rest; with whole organic raw food, supplements and herbs. I developed a health program for my brother, and he followed it. Now many years later he is still doing fine.

Throughout this time I of course was also combining foods properly when one day I received a call from my doctor's office with results of my recent blood work. The woman on the phone asked what I was doing because they rarely saw results like mine from patients many years younger. The call validated how well eating the "right" foods and combining them properly was working for me, however I fell off this program on two occasions.

The first time was during a move to a very small town in Pennsylvania where I found myself quite isolated, and became depressed. It lasted for ten long years. Years I wish I could forget. Back then I numbed the loneliness, isolation and depression with comfort foods as I struggled to maintain some degree of healthy eating. When I look back on it now, I realize it gave me time to research and garner more education in holistic nutrition, natural health therapies, and Naturopathy. I buried myself in study and food... too often, the wrong kind of food.

Eventually the poor food choices took a toll. This time, instead of helping my brother, I would have to help myself.

"IF WE COULD GIVE EVERY INDIVIDUAL THE RIGHT AMOUNT OF NOURISHMENT AND EXERCISE, NOT TOO LITTLE AND NOT TOO MUCH, WE WOULD HAVE FOUND THE SAFEST WAY TO HEALTH."

HIPPOCRATES

Our immune system has the ability to correct so many imbalances and assaults coming from many different directions. We are assaulted by chemicals in our food, in our environment, and in the air. Our medications and exposure to electromagnetic radiation from computers, cell towers, and cell phones to name a few is yet another assault on the body as it continually strives to maintain a state of stability. We can choose to support the process with wholesome organic foods eaten in the right combinations so the blood and the digestive system, both the keepers of our immunity against disease, will have the necessary nutrients available for repair.

I neglected to follow the above statement, for in that small town, I had returned to the poor dietary habits of long ago. Soon I had weight gain and a great deal of joint and muscle pain, making the simple act of walking extremely difficult. I began to notice a difference in the color of the sclera (whites) of my eyes. I became worried about pancreatic cancer since I had lost a cousin my age from this disease. I had begun bleeding out of one nostril so often I had to constantly carry a tissue. After seeing many doctors about my symptoms, I agreed to have their recommended medical tests which included a CAT scan and various blood panels to look for the cause.

Nothing was found. All the many blood tests and appointments with medical specialists and yet no diagnosis was made. One doctor recommended a prescription for anti-depressants and injections into the inflamed areas for relief of pain. I remember this time as the turning point back to health. I knew I was going downhill because I felt it. I didn't need any proof other than the extra weight I carried and the pain I was feeling. Leaving the last appointment with my doctor I remember thinking, my body wasn't letting *me* down, I let *it* down.

I had abandoned all live foods, opting instead for the typical Standard American Diet, and much of it was processed. I remember an entire year without a salad. All I wanted was chips, cheese, wine, crackers, breads, lunch meats, and lots of baked goods: anything salty, sugary and easy. What I ate was comfort food, and eating like this had to stop or I knew where it would lead.

I reluctantly took the prescriptions from the doctor for the antidepressants and remember saying I was relieved they had found nothing...at least not yet. I knew what I needed to do. Taking the prescriptions home, I tossed them in a drawer and returned to the program which had worked before when I lived in California. I also incorporated a few supplements which would help support my body's return to health, but the most important part?

I began seven weeks of eating live, whole, organic, raw food. At first I ate no cooked foods at all and nothing processed by man. The only drinks I would have were herbal tea or lemon in water. The impact was amazing. Two weeks later the pain in my legs began to subside as my weight began to change.

My healthier diet led to a release of stored toxins in my body and everything began to change. I have never found anything that has made as great an impact on my health as eating whole live foods, and now, with great results in from my recent blood work, I feel I never will.

What exactly is live or raw food? They are foods not cooked or heated over 118 degrees F so as to retain all nutrients. Fruits, vegetables, salads, raw dairy (yes, *raw* dairy) are all live foods. I have made my own fermented kefir, a pro-biotic drink, from raw goat milk for over 14 years. It is delicious. This milk is closest to mother's milk, easily digestible, alkaline and contains enzymes and numerous vitamins.

I encourage you to research the ***benefits*** of raw goat milk and make your own decision. In the book "The Blue Zones" by Dan

Buettner, the lifestyles of people in 5 zones around the world who live over 100 have many things in common from their lifestyle to their diet. One of them is their choice of drink: raw goat milk. Raw, live, whole foods not processed by man are exactly what heal the body.

Remember, in order to be classified as a food, what we eat must be able to be broken down during the process of digestion and utilized by the cells. Chemicals and additives found in so many of today's processed foods are removed through the organs of elimination, one of them being the skin. If they are not able to be removed, for whatever reason, it is likely these non food chemicals and preservatives are settling in joints or tissues in the body. I am convinced this was a major part of my pain.

Once I cleaned up my diet and my body began to detox from the processed foods, my joint and muscle pains were eliminated and have never returned. To this day, I avoid buying anything with an ingredient list containing items I do not recognize or cannot pronounce.

Foods have a time line for digestion and an order of digestion. For instance, fruits (simple carbohydrates) have a quick digestive time. First thing in the morning, they digest within an hour or two, moving to the small intestine where true digestion and absorption of nutrients occurs.

Next are complex carbohydrates, the body's source of glucose, our energy. They digest more slowly and are an excellent mid-morning or lunch time meal. The time line for digestion of the more common complex carbohydrates like potatoes, pastas, breads, and rice is around 5 hours.

Protein, on the other hand, requires a longer digestion time and is often my last meal of the day. Having this meal at least a few hours before bedtime assures it is well on the way toward digestion and will not be in the stomach in the morning. Note: Blood type A has a more difficult time digesting animal proteins as beef, chicken, fish, and eggs due to a lesser amount of hydrochloric acid in the stomach. This is *one* reason I rarely eat them. Environmental impact and treatment of animals rounds out my reasons for choosing plant proteins over animal proteins.

There has been more and more data surfacing about the benefits of choosing plant based proteins over the more commonly known animal proteins as beef, chicken, or even seafood. I find there is some confusion about plant protein. Proteins are found in small amounts in all foods. There is protein in spinach, broccoli, *and* even in fruits and vegetables. We find proteins in chia seed, hemp seed, in fact, in all seeds, as well as in nuts, and legumes as lentils. In the case of hemp seeds, they contain essential amino acids (*proteins*) needed by the body as well as essential fatty acids necessary for heath. In other words these little seeds are comparable to other proteins but *much* easier to digest. Delicious, nutritious and tasting a bit like nuts I add them to my kefir, sprinkle on salads, add to smoothies or eat them by themselves.

Not only do we get proteins from meats and eggs, we also get protein from chocolate. Listed on the label of a dark chocolate bar containing 85% cocoa you will find 4 grams of protein. In Cacao Nibs, the actual crushed chocolate nut, which by the way come from trees, there is even more protein. Cacao Nibs are also a wonderful source of fiber and a super food. If you become a label reader you will find there are many surprising sources of proteins and many of the healthiest are from easily digested plant proteins.

Fruits are my breakfast of choice first thing in the morning after my coffee. I eat enough to be full, but not stuffed. Fruits are full of vitamins, minerals and fiber and are the only food category I can eat every few hours because they digest quickly; as long as they are not eaten with other foods. As part of a healthy diet fruits help to maintain health and can reduce the risk for chronic disease.

Next, for a mid-day lunch whether at home or dining out, I might have pancakes, waffles, steel cut oatmeal, a vegetable sub or vegetable soup and green salads. All the above are excellent choices and all are carbohydrates.

Later that night, but hours before retiring, I will have my protein meal with salad, and choose various non starch vegetables such as zucchini, green beans or asparagus. I may even have a salad *and* non-starch vegetables if I am very hungry. I do not include any mild starch (beets, parsnips) or starch (breads, rice, potatoes), as these are all the wrong carbohydrates with this protein meal.

Experiment with this to see how you feel. If you do not suffer indigestion when eating high starch carbohydrates after or with a protein meal, check for weight gain. This is another sign of a miss-combined meal and it may not show up right away. If you have battled weight gain as I did all my life, you are going to be pleasantly surprised when you follow food combining. It is something you can do for life, no gimmicks, no Monday morning diets and no more guilt.

It is my hope, with the choices I give you later for various restaurants, you will begin to notice a difference in the way you feel during and after a meal.

Chapter Two
Pain Leaves and Health Returns

"Think of fruits and vegetables as an army of smart bombs ready to wipe out excess free radical damage, thus slowing the aging process; then consider how often you eat fruit."

Waking in the morning free of pain and full of energy helps keep me focused on following the program I previously described. It is simple and makes sense. No more counting calories or worrying about getting all my vitamins and minerals. Those worries are taken care of with organic whole food choices in a rainbow of colors. It is no longer even about weight loss, although that happens. When I began to eat this way, it was about gaining health; and today it is about maintaining it as I age.

The body continually cleanses and heals, but even more so at night. The entire body including the digestive system slows during sleep. If food is eaten close to retiring for the evening, more than likely, the meal is still in the stomach in the morning.

For years, one of the healthiest things I have done is drinking water with the juice of one-half lemon first thing in the morning. Lemon, an acid fruit, becomes alkaline in the body and helps to control mucus, a problem for the person with type A blood. By drinking lemon water first thing in the morning, I continue to support the cleansing that begins in the body after 8 to 12 hours without food.

This is why deep sleep is so important. The nutrients from the day's food choices provide the body with what is needed to repair itself during the healing hours of sleep. The symptoms of poor digestion are warnings from the body. If changes are not made, poorly digested meals continue to cause fermentation sending toxins back and forth through the body. The entire digestive and elimination systems become sluggish. The body is self poisoning itself as these toxins are reabsorbed over and over. This is known as auto-intoxication and can lead to disease.

Another type of damage within the body can occur from a process known as the free radical theory of aging. Briefly, free radicals are unpaired electrons within a cell and are highly unstable. The pair which loses one electron will steal an electron from a neighboring cell creating more free radical damage.

This damage occurs from the environment as well as from normal metabolism. In other words, just being alive causes free radicals. Disease itself creates free radical damage and so does drinking alcohol, smoking and even over exercising. All of these contribute to aging faster since the unstable electrons cascade into other molecules causing more cell damage. With more damage, there is more destruction to the body and we not only age quicker, we walk closer to today's lifestyle diseases.

For more information, see FREE RADICALS:A MAJOR CAUSE OF AGING AND DISEASE BY HARI SHARMA, M.D. and author of "FREEDOM FROM DISEASE."

To the rescue come antioxidants found abundantly in fruits. Fruits also contain vitamins, minerals, and enzymes which help to prevent this cellular damage. The more antioxidants we have in our bodies, the younger we feel and look and we lessen our risk for those lifestyle diseases. We become healthier. Think of fruits and vegetables as an army of smart bombs ready to wipe out excess free radical damage slowing the aging process, then consider how often you eat fruit.

I was delighted to see the government raise the dietary guidelines to include more servings of fruits and vegetables. Fruits digest quickly in the small intestine, delivering those antioxidant smart bombs to quell the excess free radical damage in the body; *and* fruits cleanse the body. I often eat two meals of fruit each morning separated by the couple of hours needed to digest each fruit.

One of the mistakes made when food combining is not enough food is eaten. In other words, if fruit is your choice for breakfast, you must allow enough time for the fruit to digest before the next meal. Thus, it is important to eat enough of it. If you have become hungry soon after eating fruit you simply did not eat enough of it.

True hunger is the body's cry for nutrition. I have at times eaten three apples and found my hunger did not return for 2 hours, a perfect digestive time for apples. Eating enough fruit provides antioxidant, nutrient dense food for a delicious, nutritious, cleansing start to the day.

In one banana there are: 3.1 grams of fiber, 1.3 grams of protein, and 0.4 grams of fat. This is an example of a complex food because all food groups are in one *food*. Contrast this with a complex *meal* (think Thanksgiving) which most people eat three times a day. The complex meal is very difficult for the body to digest, especially with the aging of the entire digestive system. This is the main reason I separate carbohydrate from protein in my meals. When I eat this way, I do not hear, feel or suffer any digestive problems.

People are sometimes confused as to what a carbohydrate is. You probably know potatoes, bread and rice are carbohydrates, but you may be surprised when I say lettuce and blueberries are also carbohydrates. In fact, all vegetables and fruits are carbohydrates. There are simple carbohydrates as fruits and the more well known complex carbohydrates as rice and potatoes.

If you are eating a food that came from an animal, it is a protein and not a carbohydrate. The meats in a typical deli sandwich are proteins just the same as the steak or fish eaten at the evening meal. That sandwich is a mis-combined meal because bread is a carbohydrate and will not digest well with protein. What would digest well, is a sandwich full of vegetables, which are all carbohydrates. If I have a sub, it is filled with vegetables

...no cheese or meats (both foods from an animal).

Carbohydrates provide us with energy and are the fuel for our bodies. This is another reason I choose to eat carbohydrates during the day when I am more active. The digestive time for carbohydrates is also much shorter than for animal protein, so consuming them midday allows plenty of time for digestion before the evening protein meal which usually contains chicken, fish or beef.

Back to lunch. If I am truly hungry after eating a carbohydrate meal mid-day, such as soup and salad, oatmeal, or pancakes; I will eat another fruit. Fruit will digest within a few hours leaving plenty of time before my evening meal. Too many meals eaten close together is often the reason for weight gain and can be an indication that the previous meal has not had enough time to digest before another meal was eaten. Your body will tell you when it is hungry.

Each one of us is different. **Begin slowly**, incorporating a few rules of food combining and see how you feel. If I am hungry before a foods digestive time is over it usually is because I did not eat enough. However it could also be due to a faster metabolism. I exercise daily and lift weights, and I am very in tune with my body. We are all different and our bodies send signals. Take time to listen.

I rarely eat beef, turkey, or chicken. Many times I am asked where I get my protein. My answer is from many different plant proteins and grains as quoina or lentils. I eat nuts, seeds, raw goat milk kefir, and eggs. I occasionally eat seafood for my blood type. One constant in my diet is greens. I eat a *lot* of greens.

Nations with the highest consumption of animal protein are some of the unhealthiest. Animals used to graze on grass and roam free. Today they are enclosed in pens and often fed genetically modified feeds such as corn or soybeans. The conditions under which the animals live often necessitate administering antibiotics to fight disease. They are sometimes given growth hormones so they will grow faster and heavier for market and produce massive amounts of milk with no resemblance to the product which the milkman delivered years ago with cream on top.

The genetically modified grains animals are fed and the medicines they are administered as in the case of antibiotics, will ultimately become part of my cells and affect my health. If I eat any animal protein I choose organic chicken, organic grass fed beef, or wild caught seafood.

Plant proteins found in fruits and vegetables are perfectly combined "complex foods" which the body can easily digest. If we don't cook fruits and vegetables they come with their own live enzymes to aid digestion. Once I adopted a plant based diet, I naturally became thinner and healthier proving Dr. D'Adamo was absolutely right. My type A blood thrives on a predominately vegetarian diet and stores meats as fat. I also found a renewed sense of energy from live foods as fruits and raw vegetables.

Before I leave the topic of protein I would like to talk about **Human Growth Hormone**, also known as HGH. Think of growth hormone as a youth elixir. What happens with age is the *ability* to secrete the hormone diminishes substantially. Proteins will enhance the release of this hormone and carbohydrates will tend to inhibit the release.

When we are young growth hormone is released at about 90% of its potential; but after a certain age, secretion begins to decline. Statistics indicate that by age 70 secretion is reduced to about 10%. Eating protein in the evening aids the body in releasing this small amount of growth hormone. Sugars and carbohydrates tend to stimulate the release of insulin which inhibits this small release of HGH and is the fat storing hormone.

This is important because HGH release is peaked at night and plays a role in repair of the body during deep sleep. If you are putting on weight while still following good food combining please examine if you are eating too many *carbohydrate* meals late at night. You may have just found the reason why you are gaining weight.

Before leaving this chapter, let's discuss desserts. I enjoy them however I am careful to choose wisely and not eat them every day. I also eat dessert only after a carbohydrate meal or by itself. Think of an Italian meal of spaghetti, salad, and bread, which are all carbohydrates. Carbohydrates digest as sugars. The dessert has a better chance of digesting with the carbohydrate meal than with a protein meal. Sugar tends to ferment protein. If you decide to eat a dessert with a protein meal and you suffer indigestion try a teaspoon of *raw* honey. Manuka honey is a superior honey with medicinal qualities that helps balance the digestive system. The live enzymes will help to mitigate the symptoms of indigestion. This is what I do when I have my 20% cheat meals and within a short amount of time, I feel amazingly better. However, remember! This still means it was a miscombined meal and the meal will not digest well no matter the relief from the *raw* honey.

Listen to your body. This works so well for me. If you do eat the dessert with the protein meal and you feel none of the symptoms of indigestion, be aware of any weight gain after the meal. It may not show up right away, but this is often another sign of a meal that has not digested properly. Important to remember because it is all about *health.*

As we continue to eat healthy foods, the body becomes healthier and rids itself of the toxic weight or poisons in the cells. Then when we make a slip and return to the old ways, we do not feel well after the meal. This is the warning the body sends when re-introducing the wrong foods and combinations. The uncomfortable symptoms return.

NORMA JEAN

KOMBUCHA

There are various opinions about the health benefits of a fermented tea called Kombucha. It is made from sweetened black tea to which a SCOBY is added. Scoby stands for...

SYMBIOTIC COLONY OF BACTERIA AND YEAST

This fermented beverage originated in the Far East over 2,000 years ago. Kombucha has B vitamins, enzymes and a long list of probiotics. It can improve digestion, increase energy and helps to detoxify the body. It can be made at home or bought in health stores as well as various grocery chains. It strengthens the immune system due to the antioxidants in the tea. Fermentation of any beverage or food, as cultured vegetables, is in itself, beneficial to the body. These fermented foods and drinks contain healthy bacteria and have been healthy additions in my diet for a very long time.

Begin with a few ounces 15 minutes before a meal to aid digestion. Enjoy it also in between a meal. One day as I offering a sample to a woman the conversation went something like this.

I already know about Kombucha, she said. My daughter came home from a trip overseas with intestinal problems. Kombucha relieved all symptoms.

I simply smiled, for I was not surprised.

WE LIVE IN A SOCIETY OF TEMPTING FOODS EVERYWHERE WE TURN. WE KNOW HOW IMPORTANT SOCIALIZATION IS FOR OUR HEALTH, ESPECIALLY OUR BRAIN. HOWEVER I FIND IT IRONIC THAT OUR HEALTH IS OFTEN DELT A BLOW BY THE FOODS SURROUNDING US, WHEN WE DO.

Chapter Three
One More Time It Works

I mentioned in a previous chapter that twice I strayed from healthy eating. When it happened the second time I had been caring for my dad who had developed Alzheimer's disease. It wasn't long before I noticed my own health was beginning to deteriorate.

Watching a family member decline from this terrible disease was so depressing, I didn't care what or when I ate. In no time at all I began putting on weight and feeling fatigued. My dad and I ate together during the time I cared for him. He loved having hamburgers and steaks but these foods are all wrong for my type A blood. Once again pain began to radiate down my right leg. Having been through this before I knew exactly where it was headed. Wrong food choices and a lack of exercise had begun the decline.

I was eating all the wrong proteins hoping to keep him from losing too much weight. I began to bake daily. It became very hard to resist the baked goods I prepared or keep from eating meats which I cooked for his blood type O. Weight gain and digestive problems were one problem, but once the pain returned it was apparent I needed to reassess how best to help my dad without my own decline. He would not have wanted that.

I hired more help for my step-mom and my brother so my dad could remain in his own home. I have made sure I can bring him to Florida if the need arises. Right now my family, along with the added help, continue to be able to care for him in his home, which of course, is best for him.

Retirement in Florida meant the end of unhealthy food choices and more time to exercise. I still return home several times each year to visit and help where I can. Before I left Pennsylvania I installed cameras in the home to be able to watch over things from afar, and four years later, although he cannot speak, he recognizes me when I return...sometimes.

So here I am in the gorgeous retirement community known as The Villages where the idea for this book finally came together. I moved here a little bit heavier needing to concentrate on myself one more time but I knew exactly what to do the second time around. Once again I had the same results I had many years ago, and I recorded the results at the USF health center here in The Villages at Lake Sumter.

Every few months I return for a body composition analysis and compare my results from the previous months. I have more than a years worth of proof on paper encouraging me to continue this journey of health.

One day, while attending a seminar in a doctors office, the idea for this book came to me. A gentleman asked the speaker, "How can I eat healthy when my wife wants to eat out every night"? I thought… 'I could answer that question'. I would say, find out your blood type and what foods you should avoid. Do not choose avoid foods from the menu and more importantly combine foods for proper digestion.

After speaking to a few small groups in The Villages I wanted to share what I had learned throughout my years of study and teach what many of us in natural health believe, myself included. Just because we age, it is not inevitable we will fall prey to lifestyle diseases. We can remain healthy if we make the correct choices each and every day toward that goal. Sometimes it is difficult to stay on the right path and we falter, as I did when taking care of my dad. The difference is now I know what and how to eat, and make necessary changes before the poor choices take me too far in the wrong direction. I do not deny myself anything but I am careful to not do it often. I know when something is amiss and I have learned to listen to the warning signs of my body.

When we understand the digestive process and how compromised it is as we age, and we begin to read ingredient lists of foods putting processed foods back on a shelf if they contain additives we do not understand or cannot pronounce; when we add more of Gods whole foods, we take back control of how we age. Therefore it is no longer scary waking up in the morning not knowing what to do. It is liberating. No diets. No more having to spend money seeking another supplement meant to make up for what food was designed to do first. Supplements are rarely the answer to correct a diet lacking healthy foods.

"LET FOOD BE THY MEDICINE
AND MEDICINE BE
THY FOOD."

HIPPOCRATES

Chapter Four
Three Things

At this time I want to state what is probably obvious but needs to be said.

When we are in charge of our own foods by buying organic. When we prepare our meals ourselves using the best fats and oils; as butter from grass fed cows, cold pressed olive oil or **raw unrefined** coconut oil. When we use *Celtic or Himalayan Salt (sodium and minerals the body can utilize without anti-caking ingredients), we have quite a different meal than one prepared by others.

*The above salts contain over 80 minerals but do not contain iodine. I obtain my iodine, which is important for thyroid health, from edible sea **vegetables** as Dulse and Arame, a species of kelp. Dulse, a purple seaweed, is my favorite and is extremely rich in nutrients. Nori is another healthy sea vegetable which is often wrapped around sushi. I like adding them to soups and salads.

I enjoy eating out as much as anyone, however most of my meals are at home. No matter where I dine, I adhere to the following three rules 90% of the time. Should you try a few of them I believe you will be pleasantly surprised at your results .

1. Separate brown from white, meaning I rarely ever eat animal proteins such as chicken, fish, turkey or beef with any breads, rice or pastas. This is the most important rule of food combining.

Almost every meal served when dining out breaks this rule. First comes the bread basket. When an order is taken I am asked if I want mashed potatoes or baked with my entree. If I order fish I usually have a choice of rice or noodles. If combining the proteins and carbohydrates above, bloating and indigestion often occurs. I separate the above and order either the protein meal or carbohydrate meal with appropriate vegetables and always add a salad to aid digestion.

2. I drink liquids (water with lemon or unsweetened tea) up to the time the meal is served.

I do not have ice in any drink as cold shocks the warmth of the stomach and hinders digestion. I drink lemon water up to 15 minutes before a meal and wait at least an hour or two after before I drink water again. Drinking large amounts of liquids during any meal can itself lead to bloating even if combining foods correctly. Try and consume water in between meals. I will sometimes enjoy one cup of coffee after a meal. If too much liquid is consumed when dining the digestive enzymes become diluted which compromises the entire digestive process.

3. In general, when it comes to fruits, eat them alone.

Eating the *small* amount of fruit found on restaurant salads is not the worst thing you could do when dining out. Fruit is more of a problem when it is eaten with a meal of animal protein as beef, chicken or fish because of the long digestive time of those proteins. Be aware of fruit on the menu of a restaurants' Signature Salad menu which usually has a choice of chicken or beef. Eating fruit with chicken or as a dessert after *any* meal is a sure fire way to ruin an otherwise properly combined meal. The fruit will ferment in the warm environment of the stomach and cause uncomfortable digestive symptoms. If I choose to eat a salad with chicken, allowable for my blood type A, I ask for the fruit to be left off the salad.

Be aware of any symptoms and how you feel when you work through the following menus as you eat for your blood type with proper food combinations. I have done my best to provide you with choices in the most popular types of restaurants. I hope you enjoy the meals.

Menu choices for each blood type, properly combined for digestion are included in Appendix A. Bon Appetite!

TEA AND COFFEE

Coffee is an antioxidant and good for us. The latest data suggests drinking more than one cup a day is even more beneficial than what was previously thought. Enjoy that morning cup of coffee. Enjoy sipping one cup slowly after a meal. At home I use organic coffee beans and a bit of coconut sugar which is a much healthier choice over processed refined white sugar. If using cream or half and half it is wise to choose organic with nothing added. When dining out there is little choice...so just enjoy.

Tea has a high level of antioxidants, vitamins and minerals. One of my favorites is Rooibos. Called 'red tea', it is a South African fermented herbal tea very high in antioxidants and slightly sweet. It is very delicious.

Green teas health benefits have been known for quite some time. Matcha green tea is powdered stone ground tea leaves. One teaspoon of matcha is like drinking 10 cups of green tea. Another favorite of mine is roasted dandelion tea. Enjoy both coffee and tea for all the health benefits they contain. I will often add a bit of stevia, an herbal sweetener, or raw honey and cinnamon to my cup of tea.

Appendix A:
Restaurant Suggestions

Food Combination Meals for Asian Restaurants

Asian Restaurant Suggestions--Blood Type A

Protein Meal- Selections Can Be Interchanged
No dessert with a protein meal
Never with rice

Appetizer	Entree Choice	Salads and Vegetables
Egg Drop Soup	Pad Thai (Chicken)	Steamed Vegetables
Seafood Soup	Broccoli with Chicken	Sauteed Green Beans
Tofu Soup	Chicken with Mixed	String Beans
Tom Yum	Vegetables	Seaweed Salad
Tofu		Ginger Salad
Pepper Salted	Vegetable Egg Foo	Thai Ruby Salad
Edamame	Young	

Carbohydrate Meal- Selections Can Be Interchanged

Appetizer	Entree Choice	Salads and Vegetables
Miso soup	Brown Rice	Spinach Garden Salad
Vegetable Soup	Sauteed Noodles	Ginger Salad
Vegetable Spring Roll	Bean Curd	Steamed Vegetables
Seaweed Soup	Fried Rice w/ Vegetables	Seaweed Salad
Clear Soup	Vegetable Delight	Snow Peas
Cucumber Roll		Garlic Bok Choy
Vietnamese Noodle Soup	Vegetable Lo Mein	Vegetable Tempura
Soba Noodle Soup w Vegetables	Moo Shu Vegetable	Sauteed Green Beans and Mushrooms
		Mixed Vegetable Curry

This restaurant usually has my favorite dessert mochi. It's ice cream inside a delectable soft rice wrap. I order it without whipped cream. The ice cream is my 20% cheat, not the whipped cream.

Asian Restaurant Suggestions--Blood Type O

Protein Meal- Selections Can Be Interchanged
No dessert with a protein meal
Never with rice

Appetizer	Entree Choice	Salads and Vegetables
Chicken Lettuce Wraps	Mongolian Beef Steamed Grouper	Broccoli Mushrooms
Vegetable Tofu/ Egg Drop Soup Pan Seared Beef Chickpea & Tomato Soup	Chicken or Vegetable Egg Foo Young Chilean Sea Bass Pad Thai with Beef Moo Shu Beef	String Beans Steamed Vegetables and Bamboo Shoots Spinach Garden Salad Garlic Baby Bok Choy

Carbohydrate Meal- Selections Can Be Interchanged

Appetizer	Entree Choice	Salads and Vegetables
Vegetable Soup Asian Sweet Potato Roll	Vegetable Tempura	Sweet Potato Mixed Vegetables
Vegetable Spring Roll Soba Noodle Soup	Vegetable Fried Rice	Seaweed Salad Ginger Salad
Sweet Potato Fries	Rice Noodles	Spinach Garden Salad
Clear Soup Cucumber Roll	Vegetable Chow Mein	Garlic Sauteed Baby Bok Choy
	Moo Shu Vegetables	Cucumber Tomato Salad

Eating rice with a protein meal is a poor combination. Take it home and enjoy it for lunch the next day with vegetables, mushrooms and a salad.

Asian Restaurant Suggestions--Blood Type B

Protein Meal- Selections Can Be Interchanged
No dessert with a protein meal
Never with rice

Appetizer	Entree Choice	Salads and Vegetables
Salmon Poppers	Mongolian Beef	Seaweed Salad
Salmon/Cucumber Roll	Beef with Mushrooms	Squid Salad House salad
Miso Soup Jalapeno Cheese Peppers	White Tuna Pepper Seared Filet	Asparagus Steamed Vegetables Bamboo Shoots
Pan Seared Beef Negimaki	Pepper Steak with Onion	Garlic Bok Choy with Mushrooms
Hot Sour Soup Egg Drop Soup	Vegetable Egg Foo Young	Bamboo Shoots & Sugar Peas

Carbohydrate Meal- Selections Can Be Interchanged

Appetizer	Entree Choice	Salads and Vegetables
Vegetable Soup	Vegetable	Seaweed Salad
Vegetable Spring Roll	Tempura Szechuan Potatoes	Ginger Salad Cabbage Slaw
Cucumber Roll	Yuxiang	Garlic Baby Bok Choy
Sweet Potato Roll	Asparagus	Sauteed Green Beans
	Sauteed Broccoli with String Beans	Asparagus Yams
	Brown Rice with Vegetables	Vegetables Ginger Chinese Cabbage

Be aware of sweet dishes and sweet sauces. Ask for sauce on the side. Ordering a salad and steamed vegetables will help digestion. Try bread pudding or sherbert for dessert. Check digestion.

Asian Restaurant Suggestions--Blood Type AB

Protein Meal- Selections Can Be Interchanged
No dessert with a protein meal
Never with rice

Appetizer	Entree Choice	Salads and Vegetables
Egg Drop Soup	Pepper Tuna	Seaweed Salad
Beef Negimaki	Tataki	Ginger Salad
Ahi Tuna with	Saki Glazed	House Salad
Wasabi	Salmon	Spinach Garden Salad
Edamame	Seared Tuna	Tuna /Seaweed Salad
Squid Salad	Spicy Tuna	Garlic Bok Choy
Vegetable Tofu Soup	Vegetable Egg	Broccoli with Garlic
Hot Sour Soup	Foo Young	Sauce

Carbohydrate Meal- Selections Can Be Interchanged

Appetizer	Entree Choice	Salads and Vegetables
Miso Soup/no Tofu	Vegetable Lo	Seaweed Salad
Vegetable Spring	Mein/Chow Mein	Sauteed Broccoli
Roll	Rice Noodles	Bean Curd
Sweet Potato Roll	with Snow Peas	Ginger Salad
Vegetable Rice Soup	Vegetables w/	Sauteed Green Beans
Hot Sour Soup	Fried Rice	with Mushrooms
Rice Vermicelli	Vegetable Pad	Saffron Brown Rice
Soup	Thai	w/Vegetables

Be careful of sweet sauces with protein meals, as sugars could cause a digestive upset if the meal begins to ferment. Try creme brulee or sherbet after the carbohydrate meal. Check digestion.

IF I WERE TO DRINK ALCOHOL, AND I DO NOT, I WOULD ENJOY A GLASS OF WINE WITH THE FOLLOWING MEALS. SIPPING ONE GLASS OF WINE WITH A MEAL IS FINE. HAVING ALCOHOL OFTEN, OR IN EXCESS, IS NOT.

Food Combination Meals for Italian Restaurants

Italian Restaurant Suggestions--Blood Type A

Protein Meal- Selections Can Be Interchanged
No dessert with a protein meal
No pasta

Appetizer	Entree Choice	Salads and Vegetables
Fried	Lily's Chicken/w Goat	Side Salad
Mozzarella	Cheese	Greek Salad with Feta
Escargot w/o	Norwegian Salmon	Cheese
Toast Points	Chicken Romano	Spinach Salad w/egg
Tuna Poke	Chicken Picatta	Brussels Sprouts
Kale Soup	Vegetable Ricotta	Spinach Kale Salad
	Cheese Lasagna	Zucchini Leeks

Carbohydrate Meal- Selections Can Be Interchanged

Appetizer	Entree Choice	Salads and Vegetables
Stuffed	Pasta with Olive	Garden Salad
Mushrooms	Oil and Garlic	Arugula Salad
Bread and Butter	Portobello	Greek Salad w/o Cheese
Onion Soup	Vegetable Stack	Swiss Chard
with Croutons	Broccoli Stromboli	Carrots Peas Green
Garlic Knots /no	without Cheese	Beans
Marinara	Pasta with Veggies	Spinach Arugula Salad
Onion Rings		Parsnip Mashed Potatoes

This blood type thrives as a vegetarian. Limit red sauce choosing occasionally. If ordering pizza try white pizza with lots of vegetables and add a salad for digestion. A *sprinkling* of Parmesan cheese should be fine. Try ricotta cheesecake for dessert.

Italian Restaurant Suggestions--Blood Type O

Protein Meal- Selections Can Be Interchanged
No dessert with a protein meal
No pasta

Appetizer	Entree Choice	Salads and Vegetables
Shrimp Cocktail	Chicken Veal or	Mozzarella, Tomato
Crab Cake	Salmon Piccata	and Basil Salad
Mussels Marinara	Veal Marsala	Garden Salad
Fried Mozzarella	Red Snapper	Greek Salad with
with Marinara	Shrimp Scampi	Cheese w/o croutons
Italian Wedding	Shrimp Caprese	Arugula Salad
Soup /no Noodles	Gluten Free Pasta	Sauteed Kale
	Seared Scallop Salad	Zucchini
	Sirloin Steak Salad	Asparagus
		Green Beans

Carbohydrate Meal- Selections Can Be Interchanged

Appetizer	Entree Choice	Salads and Vegetables
Vegetable Soup	Beans and Broccoli	Spinach Salad w/o Egg
Broccoli Rabe	Gluten-Free Pizza	Romaine Salad
Gluten-Free	with Red Sauce	Broccoli
Bread and Butter	Gluten-Free	Yams
Onion Rings	Spaghetti with Red	Zucchini
Fried Artichoke	Sauce	Parsnip Mashed Potato

This blood type should avoid gluten. If ordering *regular* pizza with *gluten*, order a thin crust with a *sprinkling* of Parmesan cheese. Order a side salad to aid digestion.

Italian Restaurant Suggestions--Blood Type B

Protein Meal- Selections Can Be Interchanged
No dessert with a protein meal
No pasta

Appetizer	Entree Choice	Salads and Vegetables
Cheddar Colby	Lamb Shanks with	Garden Salad
Brie Edam Gouda	Mushrooms	Greek Salad with
Cheese Plate	Veal Piccata	Cheese w/o croutons
Jalapeno Poppers	Cod	Spinach Salad
Pepper Edamame	Sole	Green Beans
Onion Soup	Mahimahi	Brussels Sprouts
Vegetable Soup	Halibut	Sauteed Kale
Bean Soup	Eggplant Parmesan	Carrots
	no Marinara Sauce	Cauliflower
		Collard Greens

Carbohydrate Meal- Selections Can Be Interchanged

Appetizer	Entree Choice	Salads and Vegetables
Potato Soup	Spinach Pasta	Spinach Salad w/o Egg
Stuffed	Fried Eggplant	Arugula Salad/Yams
Mushrooms	Pasta with Olive Oil	Beets Carrots Broccoli
Garlic Knots	and Vegetables	Cauliflower Zucchini
Swt/Potato Fries	Potato Gnocchi	Roasted Root Veggies

Fermented dairy (yogurt/kefir) are healthy choices containing healthy bacteria for the immune system.

Italian Restaurant Suggestions--Blood Type AB

Protein Meal- Selections Can Be Interchanged
No dessert with a protein meal
No pasta

Appetizer	Entree Choice	Salads and Vegetables
Ahi Tuna with Wasabi	Scallops Salmon	Garden Salad Spinach Salad
Mussels in White Sauce Calamari	Mahimahi Meatballs with Marinara Sauce	Greek Salad w/Feta Grilled Asparagus Zucchini
Escargot w/o Toast Points Fried Mozzarella	Eggplant Parmesan with Marinara Sauce	Broccoli Sauteed Kale Snow Peas

Carbohydrate Meal- Selections Can Be Interchanged

Appetizer	Entree Choice	Salads and Vegetables
Bread with Butter Stuffed Mushrooms Bruschetta Garlic Knots with Marinara Sauce	Vegetarian Ravioli Gnocchi with Red Sauce Spaghetti with Red Sauce w/o Meat Rigatoni a la Vodka	Spring Mix Salad Spinach Salad w/o egg Asparagus Sweet Potatoes Sauteed Green Beans with Mushrooms

A healthy choice for this blood type is seafood. Cultured or fermented dairy (yogurt/kefir) are healthy choices; be sure there is no added sugar. Try frozen yogurt for dessert or dark chocolate.

Food Combination Meals for Mexican Restaurants

Mexican Restaurant Suggestions--Blood Type A

Protein Meal- Selections Can Be Interchanged
No dessert with a protein meal
No chips salsas or wraps

Appetizer	Entree Choice	Salads and Vegetables
Black Bean Dip	Chile Relleno	Side Salad
With Vegetables	Grilled Chicken	Garden Salad
Black Bean Soup	Huevos Rancheros	Romaine Salad
Fiesta Wings	Chicken Fajitas	Sauteed Vegetables

Carbohydrate Meal- Selections Can Be Interchanged

Appetizer	Entree Choice	Salads and Vegetables
Nachos w/o Salsa	Potato Burrito	Romaine Salad
Baja Enchilada	Spinach Quesadilla	Re-fried Beans
Soup	Butternut Squash	Rice/ Fried Rice
Black Bean Soup	Enchiladas	Tossed Salad
Tablouleh with	Vegetable Fajitas	Garden Salad *without*
Corn Chips or	Zucchini Burrito w/o	Tomatoes
Pita Chips	Cheese	

No salsa or tomatoes. Chips can be eaten alone in the carbohydrate meal. A favorite of mine is the protein cheese stuffed Poblano pepper. Wraps served with beef or chicken proteins are all poor combinations for Type A. Enjoy Mexican food as your 20% meal and eat well the other 80%. Beans contain protein and starch digesting for some as either. I have added them to both meals.

Mexican Restaurant Suggestions--Blood Type O

Protein Meal- Selections Can Be Interchanged
No dessert with a protein meal
No chips corn or flour wraps

Appetizer	Entree Choice	Salads and Vegetables
Bean Dip	Chile Relleno with	Romaine Salad with
Hummus	Beef or Cheese	Tomatoes
Tomatillo Dip with	Shrimp Mexican	Side Salad with
Vegetables	Style	Tomatoes
Baja Enchilada	Huevos Rancheros	Pinto Beans
Soup	Shrimp Al Mojo in	Mexican Chopped
Chili w/Cheese	Butter Sauce	Salads
Lime Soup	Fried Tofu	Grilled Onions, Peppers,
w/Chicken	Aztec Salad with	and Mushrooms
Fiesta Wings	Chicken	Grilled Vegetables

Carbohydrate Meals- Selections Can Be Interchanged
No corn or flour wraps for type O.

Appetizer	Entree Choice	Salads and Vegetables
Roasted Jalapeno	Vegetarian Stack	Side Vegetarian Salad
Garlic Salsa with	Vegetable Poblano	Re-fried Beans
Rice Nachos	Pepper	Mexican Rice
	(Chile Relleno)	Sauteed Vegetables

Flour and corn wraps are staples in Mexican restaurants and neither are good for Type O. Use the 20% rule as you make choices. Beans are good sources of protein and they contain carbohydrates. Do your own research to see which is best for your digestion.

Mexican Restaurant Suggestions--Blood Type B

Protein Meal- Selections Can Be Interchanged
No dessert with a protein meal
Choose beef instead of chicken
No chips corn or flour wraps

Appetizer	Entree Choice	Salads and Vegetables
Jalapeno Peppers with Cheese	Huevos Rancheros Mexican Beef stew	Romaine Salad Iceberg Salad
Poblano Pepper soup/ *no* chicken	Seafood -*No* Shellfish	Chopped Salad *no* Tomatoes
	Beef Taco Salad w/o Tortilla Chips or Taco Shell Bowl	Re-fried Beans and Rice

Carbohydrate Meal- Selections Can Be Interchanged
Corn and flour wraps are avoids so try and limit them

Appetizer	Entree Choice	Salads and Vegetables
Tortilla Soup with *Rice* Chips Tabbouleh with *Rice* Chips Poblano Pepper Soup /no Chicken Vegetable Soup	Spinach Enchiladas w/o Cheese Rice and Beans Steak Fajita w/Onions and Peppers	Chopped Salad Romaine Salad Peppers Sauteed with Mushrooms and Onions Re-fried Beans Mexican Rice with Sauteed Vegetables

This is a difficult menu due to corn or flour in tortilla wraps and chips. Beans will pose the biggest challenge because beans can digest for some as a protein and for others as a carbohydrate. If you eat them with animal protein, be aware of your digestion.

Mexican Restaurant Suggestions--Blood Type AB

Protein Meal- Selections Can Be Interchanged
No dessert with a protein meal
No corn chips   No flour or corn wraps

Appetizer	Entree Choice	Salads and Vegetables
Gouda Cheese Soup	Steak Fajitas /no Wraps	Spinach Salad Romaine Salad
Green Lentil Soup	eat filling only	Iceberg Wedge
Mex.Lentil Soup	Garden Salad with	Mushrooms &
Pumpkin Soup	Grilled Beef	Grilled Vegetables
Chili w/Cheese	Re-fried Beans	
Mex/Tomato Soup		

Carbohydrate Meal- Selections Can Be Interchanged
Flour Wraps only in Carbohydrate Meal.

Appetizer	Entree Choice	Salads and Vegetables
Rice Chips and Salsa Mexican Vegetable Soup	Spinach and Mushroom Enchilada or Spinach Burrito	Chopped Side Salad Carrot/Cabbage Slaw Sauteed Vegetables
Bean Dip with Rice Chips	Vegetable Fajitas Vegetable Quesadilla w/o Cheese	Saffron Brown Rice
Tabbouleh and Rice Chips	Rice/Re-Fried Beans	Ensalada Grande

This is a difficult menu because beans are both a protein and starch food. See which works best for your digestion. Corn or flour tortilla wraps served with beef or chicken meals are mis-combined. This may be your 20% exception to proper food combining. Eat what you enjoy and choose carefully the other 80% of the time.

HIS FOODS

Food Combination Meals for Steak and Seafood Restaurants

Steak /Seafood Restaurant Suggestions--Blood Type A

Protein Meal- Selections Can Be Interchanged
No dessert with a protein meal

Appetizer	Entree Choice	Salads and Vegetables
Escargot w/o Toast Points	Red Snapper	Garden Salad
Cheddar Stuffed Mushrooms	Talapia with Mushrooms	Greek Salad with Feta
French Onion or Black Bean Soup	Pesto Chicken	Spinach Salad with Egg
	Sole	Mixed Vegetables
	Haddock	Asparagus
Ahi Tuna Sashimi	Monkfish	Sauteed Mushrooms and Onions
Fried Artichokes	Grilled Mahimahi	

Carbohydrate Meal- Selections Can Be Interchanged
No fish steak or chicken

Appetizer	Entree Choice	Salads and Vegetables
Bread Sticks	Seasoned Rice w/ Vegetables	Spinach Salad w/o Egg
Bread and Butter		Iceberg Wedge
Dipping Oil with Bread	Pasta with Olive Oil Garlic & Vegetables	Side House Salad
		Carrots
Kettle Chips	Lemon Pesto	Green Beans
Mushroom Soup	Fettuccini	Beets
Ahi Tuna		Turnips

Blood Type A is especially suited to a vegetarian diet with lots of greens . Fish is a healthier choice over meats of any kind. Type A can tolerate a bit of white flour so try cake for dessert after a carbohydrate meal. Be aware of digestion. Frozen yogurt is another good choice.

<u>Steak/Seafood Restaurant Suggestions--Blood Type O</u>

<u>Protein Meal</u>- Selections Can Be Interchanged
No dessert with a protein meal

Appetizer	Entree Choice	Salads and Vegetables
Chicken Wings	Prime Rib/ Fillet	Garden Salad
Crab Stuffed	Steak	Spinach Salad
Mushrooms	Meatloaf	Spring Mix Salad
French Onion	Mahimahi	Asparagus
Soup /no	Shrimp	Green Beans
Croutons	Halibut	Leeks
Shrimp Cake	Lobster	Swiss Chard
Shrimp Cocktail	Tuna Salad	Sauteed Mushrooms and
Crab Cake	Grilled Salmon	Onions
Steamed Clams	Snapper	Zucchini Broccoli

<u>Carbohydrate Meal</u>- Selections Can Be Interchanged
No fish steak or chicken

Appetizer	Entree Choice	Salads and Vegetables
Onion Soup w/o	Vegetable Soup	Iceberg Wedge Salad
Cheese	Seasoned Rice	Spinach Salad
w/ Croutons	with Vegetables	Carrots
Cuban Black Bean	Sweet Potato	Asparagus Zucchini
Soup	Roasted Root	Green Beans
Onion Rings	Vegetables	

Beans digest as either protein or carbohydrate. Check digestion.

Grass fed beef and cold water fish are healthier choices so opt for them if they are offered on a menu. Salads are important for digestion with the type O acidic digestive system. Try dark chocolate desserts w/o dairy. No desserts with flour. A flour less chocolate cake would be fine with the carbohydrate meal.

Steak/Seafood Restaurant Suggestions--Blood Type B

Protein Meal- Selections Can Be Interchanged
No dessert with a protein meal

Appetizer	Entree Choice	Salads and Vegetables
Cheddar Stuffed Mushrooms	Rosemary/ Mushroom Filet	Spinach Brie Salad Greek Salad with Feta
Jalapeno Poppers Onion Soup with Cheese w/o Croutons	Teriyaki Steak Medallions Prime Rib Roasted Lamb	Chopped Salad w/o Croutons Kale Zucchini
Brie Gouda Edam	Halibut	All Peppers
Mushroom Brie Soup	Catfish	Roasted Peppers with Mushrooms and Onions

Carbohydrate Meal- Selections Can Be Interchanged
No fish steak or chicken

Appetizer	Entree Choice	Salads and Vegetables
Fried artichoke Fried Onion Rings	Baked Navy Beans /Yams	House Salad Spinach Salad /no Egg
Baked Pretzel Sticks Bread with Butter	Semolina Pasta Brown Rice Potato w/butter	Side Salad Broccoli Rapini Yellow squash

Try to limit corn and tomatoes. They are an avoid food for type B. Be very careful of chicken for it is a problem in this blood type and should be eliminated from the diet. Choose turkey instead. For Dessert after the carbohydrate meal try cheesecake or frozen yogurt.

Steak/Seafood Restaurant Suggestions-Blood Type AB

Protein Meal-Selections Can Be Interchanged
No dessert with a protein meal

Appetizer	Entree Choice	Salads and Vegetables
Calamari w/ Wasabi	Rack of Lamb Salmon	Garden Salad Spinach Salad with Egg
Escargot w/o Toast Points	Red Snapper Mussels/Sardines	Greek Salad with Feta String Beans Almondine
Onion Soup w/o Croutons Broccoli Cheese Soup	Sole Scallops Cod Mahimahi Ahi Tuna	Cauliflower Mashed Potatoes Peas Zucchini Kale Eggplant

Carbohydrate Meal- Selections Can Be Interchanged
No fish steak or chicken

Appetizer	Entree Choice	Salads and Vegetables
Bread with Butter Onion Soup with Croutons	Potato Soup w/o cheese Wild Rice Pilaf	Garden Salad Spinach Salad no egg Fried Eggplant
Onion Rings Sweet Potato Fries	Baked Potato with Butter	Spinach Beets Turnips Carrots
Vegetable Soup Tomato Basil Soup French Fries	Sweet Potato with Honey Butter	Broccoli Kale Parsnip Mashed Potatoes Cauliflower Carrots Snow Peas Zucchini

Try rice or quinoa pasta when cooking at home. Rice is better than most pastas for Type AB. Try rice pudding, ricotta cheesecake, or yogurt for dessert. Lucky you can also try cheesecake for dessert.

HIS FOODS

Appendix B:
Food Combining

The lists on the following pages will show in general terms how you can combine foods that you select from the menu in such a way that digestion may be made easy.

MEALS WITH PROTEIN

If you choose an animal protein meal, eat plenty of salad greens and vegetables. No pasta, bread, or other starches allowed. Combining greens with protein will shorten digestive time due to the live enzymes in salads. For best digestion, select one food from either animal or starch protein.

Protein Starch

Beans
Dry Peas
Soy Beans
Quinoa
Tofu

Animal Protein

Egg
Fowl
Meat
Seafood
Veal/ Lamb

Non Starch /Green Vegetables

Artichoke	Celery	Onion
Asparagus	Collards	Peas,fresh
Beet Tops	Cucumber	Radish
Bamboo shoots	Dandelion	Parsley
Bell Pepper	Eggplant	Spinach
Bok Choy	Garlic	Sprouts
Broccoli	Green Beans	Swiss Chard
Brussels Sprout	Kale	Watercress
Cabbage	Lettuce (all)	Zucchini
Cauliflower	Mushroom	

Fats

Ghee/Butter- from grass fed cows -Olive oil
Unrefined Coconut Oil

Olive oil with lemon is a healthy dressing for salads. Lemon will aid the digestion of fat and the greens will add enzymes which help to shorten the digestive time of the meal.

MEALS WITH CARBOHYDRATES

If you want pasta, bread, rice, potatoes, and maybe a dessert, then eat these with lots of salad greens and vegetables. No protein in this meal. It should digest in 3 to 5 hours.

Mild starch

Beet
Carrot
Parsnip
Turnip
Oatmeal
Quinoa

Starch

Bread   Pasta
Cereal   Peanut (raw)
Corn   Popcorn
Cracker   Potato
Pumpkin   Jicama
Lima Bean   Rice

Non Starch/ Green Vegetables

Artichoke   Celery   Onions
Asparagus   Collards   Peas, fresh
Beet Tops   Cucumber   Radish
Bamboo shoots   Dandelion   Parsley
Bell Pepper   Eggplant   Spinach
Bok Choy   Garlic   Sprouts
Broccoli   Green Beans   Swiss Chard
Brussels Sprout   Kale   Watercress
Cabbage   Lettuce (all)   Zucchini
Cauliflower   Mushroom

Fats

Ghee/Butter- from grass fed cows-Olive oil

Unrefined Coconut Oil

Olive oil with lemon is a healthy dressing for salads. Lemon will aid the digestion of fat and the greens will add enzymes which help to shorten the digestive time of the meal.

If hungry for cheese, avocado, nuts, olives or sour cream, then this is your choice. Loading up on salad greens and vegetables is not only healthier, it shortens the digestive time of the meal due to the live enzymes in greens.

Protein Fat

Avocado
Cheese
Nuts
Olives
Seeds
Sour Cream
Yogurt(not fat free)

Non Starch /Green Vegetables

Artichoke	Celery	Onions
Asparagus	Collards	Peas, fresh
Beet Tops	Cucumber	Radish
Bamboo shoots	Dandelion	Parsley
Bell Pepper	Eggplant	Spinach
Bok Choy	Garlic	Sprouts
Broccoli	Green Beans	Swiss Chard
Brussels Sprout	Kale	Watercress
Cabbage	Lettuce (all)	Zucchini
Cauliflower	Mushroom	

Fats

Ghee/Butter- from grass fed cows-Olive oil

Unrefined Coconut Oil

Olive oil with lemon is a healthy dressing for salads. Lemon will aid the digestion of fat and the greens will add enzymes which help to shorten the digestive time of the meal.

Notes

Dining at Home

Symptoms

Notes

Dining in Restaurants

Symptoms

NORMA JEAN

Appendix C:
Dermascope Article

The following is reprinted from <u>Dermascope</u>,
November 2007.

Nutrition and Skin Care
       By: Norma Jean

Five years after writing my first article on how the digestive
system impacts skin, I find that very little has changed in how
those of us within the skin industry are educating clients. In fact, I
find very little education being done at all, and I wonder why. Do
not misunderstand me, please. Most of us do educate about the
products and treatments used in client care, but when our clients
walk away from us, what understanding does a client have of the
nutrition needed for great skin? It is not yester-year when skin
care consisted of cleansers, toners, and moisturizers. It is much
different today, and turning away from what is ultimately going to
have a large impact in this industry is not good business. Putting it
on the back burner until another time may leave you wishing you
had begun long ago to understand the importance of nutrition in
skin care.

Upon publication of my article in 2002, I received many e-mails
from those in the industry but many more from the public, wanting
to know more about the process known as glycation that
contributes to wrinkling and sagging of the skin. This glycation
that occurs in the body from a process caused by too many wrong
dietary choices, has not only a detrimental effect on the skin, but
can cause many problems in the body as well. As aestheticians, we
are concerned mainly about the skin as it pertains to what is seen
on the outside, but should we consider more?

My concern is this: If we do not understand how this organ is
affected by daily dietary choices, then how can we deliver our best
work? We ultimately will lose clients. Nothing affects the skin
more, other than a skilled plastic surgeon, than the food choices
clients make daily. Even in the case of the plastic surgeon, his
mastery with facial surgery can be enhanced when his clients are
taught how to keep the skin from glycation through proper
nutritional choices. As aestheticians, how many of us think about
approaching plastic surgeons for a position that would entail

enhancing the results of their work through nutritional education for their clients? If surgeons' clients could be taught how to keep that new face lift from sagging and wrinkling after spending thousands to achieve a younger look, I would think that the surgeon and indeed the client would benefit from such a service during post-operative care.

The impact of how the nutrients from our food choices are digested and ultimately delivered to the cells and body during the process of digestion determines our state of health. This includes the skin. Eating a diet high in white anything, as in processed foods, potato chips, cookies, baked potatoes, candy, or even white breads or pastas, impacts not only the body but the skin. What occurs is a process known as inflammation. In fact many feel this inflammation as shoes get tighter or a waist band needs to be loosened. This occurs in every cell and affects every organ. In fact, inflammation is a contributing factor in most major diseases today including diabetes, cancer, and you bet... obesity.

Nutrition and Inflammation Within

Beautiful skin: that catch phrase you hear everywhere, and often see in plastic surgery, dermatology, or spa ads. It often states, "beautiful skin... *from within*." Many times, when I delve deeper into that ad, or call, I find that what they are selling are supplements. It's a wise addition to every skin program. However, I wonder how much time is spent in truly educating that client about the choices she makes daily in her foods. This is important because the internal impact from her dietary choices will ultimately be seen externally in many different ways, one of them being wrinkling. I believe too many of us do not consider education about nutrition important. However, if dietary choices are causing inflammation and glycation, we have a situation as skin professionals, where we are treating problems topically that should and could be tackled at the source, In other words, prevent the inflammation internally (cellular level) through proper nutritional choices, before it occurs and is seen externally (skin), or it becomes more difficult to treat.

Within is often overused. It is not just how well our products are working topically; it means that we must affect deep within the dermis, within each cell, nutrient rich cellular replication, so that when those cells come to the surface, they contribute to a more youthful appearance. We in fact need to teach our clients, through nutritional education, how to keep that wrinkling and sagging from occurring at the point of origin deep in the cell, so that our products do the very best they can for the client.

The choices in lifestyle, as well as dietary choices the client makes, ultimately impact her skin for months, and even years later. Helping clients *understand* the impact these choices will have on skin will give them a sense of being in control of the results.

<u>Moving On to Do More</u>
Again, with every dietary choice made, we either contribute to a healthy cellular division or one that is compromised. A topical cream or treatment can stimulate cellular exfoliation, or collagen, but the desired effect will be far superior if that client understands how excess circulating sugar (bad), or antioxidants (good), impact that skin from within, through nutritional choices. Achieving that goal is something every aesthetician who is concerned with client retention should understand, for it is the point of difference. It is that edge that separates us within the industry into either looking at the skin topically or understanding what is going on from within.

Go beyond what you have learned about treatments and products, and seek out the courses about nutrition so that you can better affect the health of not just the skin, but the body as well, for the body will go along for the ride; a ride to better health, that occurs through understanding the skin as an organ. Making a difference in the skin of the client through understanding nutrition is a choice to make a difference in the body. That is because what is seen on the skin (inflammation, glycation, hyper-pigmentation, even wrinkling), is often what is occurring on a much deeper level within other organs of the body. In other words, healthy skin, healthy body.

Looking at an Age Old Problem in a Different Light

Hyper-pigmentation, that unsightly browning seen in the epidermis, began long ago. We know one contributing factor is the sun, which by the way, is an inflammatory response topically! We know how quickly our clients want results when it comes to those unsightly brown spots. Pointing out to the client how she is contributing to this process of hyper-pigmentation by causing an inflammatory response within the body from her dietary choices gives her the tools necessary to make correct food choices. There is less need for stronger products because tackling a problem at the source makes it easier to resolve. In fact, along with the clients' sunscreen, we can often get great results using milder products along with nutritional advice to prevent the process that creates the hyper-pigmentation in the first place. That is a recipe for less stress for us and great results for the client.

When we sell clients procedures that cost hundreds and sometimes thousands of dollars, we must ask ourselves if there is something else we need to be doing to give our clients the best in care. That something is not just knowledge; it is understanding. When they walk out of that treatment room, we want them to leave with something different that sets us apart from others out there. It is one thing to share knowledge, but another entirely for that knowledge to be understood. I find that people often know (knowledge) what to do, but often are not sure of how to apply that knowledge for results once they leave (understand).

Follow up and Understanding

How many of us simply sell a treatment package, allow a client to leave with hundreds of dollars in products, and never see that client again? What have we sent the client home with that would have her returning for more? In fact, are the treatments or products even working as they should for that client, for if our products do not give her satisfaction, she will have many other choices. Consider also, if clients do not realize the impact nutritional choices have on skin, some may begin to complain that products are not working. They may circumvent all the good that the treatments and products may be trying to accomplish due to wrong choices in foods.

Consider this one fact: The blood can only hold a few teaspoons of "sugar" at a time. This includes potatoes, rice, and of course that all delicious candy bar. A little fact here is that a potato will send more circulating sugar into the body as it is digested than an Almond Joy bar and that is because that candy bar has almonds. Almonds contain the good fats that help to slow the digestion of the sugar which allows a lower glycemic response in the body. This is good, but a better option would be eating the almonds alone. Remember that when there is excess circulating sugar, there is more inflammation, which means more insulin is secreted by the pancreas. How that impacts us as aestheticians is that when excess circulating sugar does occur through diet, the response by the body is an attack on the collagen and elastin in the skin and that causes wrinkles and sagging.

A New "Age" for Skin

Some of us may wonder how we can speak to the needs of the skin concerning nutrition, when it is such a vast unknown area to many. Our licenses say aestheticians, not dieticians. Yet, years ago, supplements came into play within the skin care industry. I remember being overwhelmed trying to decide which ones to buy or advise my clients on. Some of you may feel that same sense of where to begin and what to learn? There are so many supplements at the trade shows. Many of us have money tied up in supplements that no one buys, because we do know of the importance (knowledge), but we do not understand how to apply it. In fact, how many of you have moved away from this important component in skin care altogether?

Supplements are just what they are… a supplement …to our diet! We were designed to obtain our nutrition from foods as they are digested. What we all have in common is the digestive system. Unless we have been altered through surgery, that system responsible for our health, the health of all our organs, skin included, works the same for all of us. Understanding how that system works, learning how food choices impact this system and ultimately the skin, makes a lot more sense than trying to decipher what nutritional supplements to sell, to correct a skin problem that may or may not be helped by a supplement we know little about.

I can hear it now. 'As an aesthetician, why should this concern me?' The statistics out there point to a huge flood into the marketplace of people in their 60's (baby boomers) that have made the rounds of treatments, have dozens of products lining their shelves, and have had enough of skin care 101. Many of those treatments and products may or may not have worked well and with age many are now wondering what to do. This well-educated client is now even realizing that less is more... less products, less treatments. Where does that leave us, or the client? The skin is now sagging and more wrinkled than ever before. With all the new information out there about nutrition's impact on skin, the educated client knows there is a piece of the puzzle missing. Where will that person go for answers? Why not go to us?

Let's realize that our client's concern is skin. Skin is an organ of the body, and what is put into that body affects that skin both inside and out. This fact alone is enough for those that work within our industry that truly care about delivering the best in skin care, to move toward the education needed to better serve clients, or those clients may be lost to a more educated aesthetician.

Be the face of the changing skin care professional whether you work in a spa, for yourself, or a doctor. An aesthetician who is not only the best in providing treatments and products, but one that truly educates the client to understanding that the way to beautiful skin on the outside does come from understanding how the body works within. You will not only change your client's skin, you will see a change in the health of the client as well, and that is a feeling unlike any other.

Appendix D:
The Dangers in Our Foods

If our grandparents could walk through our super markets today, do you think they would wonder about the many boxes and cans lining the store shelves? I can just imagine my grandmother's reaction as I explain what they contain. I would tell her this is progress; but there is little good I could say beyond that. Processed foods today have so many additives, chemicals and preservatives that it is hard to keep abreast of the latest. Even if she could understand these additives to the foods, she would certainly ask "Why so many"?

Foods are meant to be broken down during the process of digestion to fuel our body and to keep us healthy. These additives are not foods and they serve no purpose except to excite the taste buds, making us eat more or, even worse, causing cells in our brains to die.

Dr. Russell L. Blaylock, M.D. warned of cell death in the brain from common excitotoxins known as MSG and aspartame. In his opinion, backed with scientific studies, he wrote that these additives posed a serious danger to neurological health. Thinking of my dad, now suffering with Alzheimer's, I remember the statistics from alz.org about the increase of this disease: "every 67 seconds someone in the United States develops Alzheimer's."

These chemicals and additives have no place in our diets...not if we want to remain healthy. In Dr. Blaylock's book "Excitotoxins: The Taste that Kills," some of the foods he lists which frequently contain MSG are stock, flavorings, seasonings, bouillon, broth, natural flavorings, and spices. Other additives that may contain MSG and excitotoxins are whey protein isolate, soy protein isolate and an additive called carrageenan.

The additive carrageenan is found in many foods today, including some almond and coconut milk as well as many dairy creams and yogurts. Dr. Blaylock's second book "Health and Nutrition Secrets that can Save Your Life" states "The common food additive carrageenan is known to trigger powerful inflammation when injected or even rubbed on the skin..."

Carrageenan is known to affect people with digestive issues, so trying to avoid this excitotoxin may help to alleviate some digestive symptoms. Chemicals and preservatives used in processing foods today are so numerous, I simply do not buy anything containing ingredients I cannot pronounce and recognize. There are obesogens that alter our weight control system, thereby increasing our fat cells. The best known is high fructose corn syrup (HFC) which encourages the body to store fat. The HFCs also shut down the hormone in the brain known as leptin. Leptin lets us know when we are full!

It reminds me of the Dr. Oz television show when he had an audience member hold up the omentum. This organ extends from the stomach, hangs in front of the intestine, and extends to the liver. It holds a storehouse of chemicals and is where internal body fat is stored. This is why belly fat is so dangerous. During stress, the fat storing hormone cortisol increases the size of this organ. A healthy diet along with exercise reduces the size of the omentum and also reduces the chemicals which impact the body in a negative way.

Then there are the endocrine disruptors known as Xenoestrogens, - chemicals which alter the normal function of hormones. They are found in our personal care products, in water, in plastics, and *sprayed on our foods*.

Lastly, consider the Genetically Modified Foods which contain genetically modified organisms (GMOs). From WEB M.D. "Are bio tech foods safe to eat?..."crops that have been modified in the laboratory to enhance desired traits such as resistance to herbicides or to improve nutritional content...this science, like any other, has no guarantees." That was enough for me. What are the benefits stated in the article? Increased pest and disease resistance, drought tolerance, and increased food supply. What is the impact of these GMOs? It is thought they damage the small intestine by altering our gut bacteria, creating inflammation. The European Union (EU) considers Genetically Modified Foods to be <u>Frankenfoods</u> and its position is "keep them out".

The labeling system in our country is considered by many to be flawed since most consumers do not know they are eating GMOs. If companies are labeling a food with "No GMO", they are generally doing so on their own as there are no federal or state regulations. This is another reason to buy organic and in so doing, avoid genetically modified foods.

Food should be consumed without alteration and processing by Man. If we believe, as Hippocrates stated so long ago, "Let food be thy medicine and medicine be thy food," then food must be able to be digested and used by the cells of the body.

The digestive process is taxing enough on the organs, especially as we age. Foods with excitotoxins, obesogens, xenoestrogens, chemicals, and preservatives increase the burden on the body during digestion. Reading labels will be an eye-opener if you have never done it before.

God's whole foods have none of the above until they are processed and refined by Man.

TO WALK AWAY FROM A CROWD AND DO WHAT IS
BEST FOR OUR HEALTH IS NOT OFTEN EASY, HOWEVER
THE REWARDS CAN BE MANY.

Appendix E:
Testimonials

When I decided to take Norma Jean's class at the Lifelong Learning College, "Food Combinations and Blood Type Diet's effect on Weight, Health and Skin", it was a life changer for me. I am just like many others who have tried to diet, unsuccessfully. In class, I learned how to eat nutritiously; combining my foods properly for my blood type, but also making smarter choices.

Norma Jean teaches from the heart because she wants to make a difference in as many people as possible and she is doing it not for her, but for others.

So here today, as a result of eating healthier and now conscious of food combining, I lost 6 pounds and 3 inches off my waist in 3 weeks. I always had energy, but I have even more now. With just this little bit of time, I changed my attitude towards foods. I changed my old habits for a better me. I am 65 and used to think as I got older it would be more difficult to be well. I now think age is often used as an excuse. I am accomplishing my goals.

So in ending, let me quote from "She Cannot Win Anymore"

> by B. Pfiester

> I will beat her. I will train harder. I will eat cleaner.
> I know her weaknesses. I know her strengths. I've lost to her before. But not this time. She is going down. I have the advantage because I know her well. She is the old me.

Thank you Norma Jean, you're the "BEST."

> June P.
> The Villages, FL.

February 3, 2015

Norma Jean,

I wanted to tell you about my results from my recent physical with my doctor. My triglycerides in October 2014 were 200 and now they are down to 88 four months later. All other numbers were down as well with a loss of 18 pounds since October 15th. The doctor was very pleased, as was I. I am still working on loosing 18 pounds more.

I have been staying pretty true to the information from your class. Lots of "raw" food, chicken and fish. I feel very good.

I always wanted to loose weight, to look better and some what feel better but I remember you saying, it is about being healthier, and living longer.

Thank you so much Norma Jean. I feel very blessed to get the results I've gotten.

> David P.
> The Villages, FL.

IT IS NOT INEVITABLE THAT I WILL INHERIT THE DISEASES OF MY PARENTS. IN ORDER TO CHANGE THE PROBABILITY OF THAT OUTCOME, I CHANGED THE BEHAVIORS.

Appendix F:
Glossary

Agglutination: A process in which the body targets proteins in a food which are wrong for a particular blood type and begins to clump them together in an effort to eliminate them. (Chapter 1)

Aesthetician: Licensed Skin care specialist who treats a wide variety of skin issues concentrating on the epidermis or outer layer of the skin. (Chapter 1)

Antioxidants: An antioxidant is a molecule that inhibits the oxidation of other molecules. Oxidation is a chemical reaction producing free radicals. In turn, these free radicals can start chain reactions. When the chain reaction occurs in a cell, it can cause damage or death to the cell. Antioxidants terminate these chain reactions. They are found in fruits and vegetables. (Chapter 2)

Carbohydrate: The body's basic source of energy and one of the classes of nutrients needed by the body. Found in certain foods (such as bread, rice, and potatoes) they provide your body with heat and energy. (Chapter 2)

Carrageenan: A food additive made from seaweed, and is known to produce intense inflammatory reactions in the body. Carrageenan is a common additive used today as a thickener in many foods including dairy. (Appendix D)

Celtic sea salt: No refining, oven drying or chemical additives are added to this moist unrefined sea salt found off the coastal areas of France. Light gray in color this salt contains 82 vital trace minerals. (Chapter 4)

Chia Seed: A nutritional dense seed with fiber protein and omega 3 fatty acids. Chia seeds can absorb up to 15 times their weight in water helping regulate body fluid and retain electrolytes. (Chapter 1)

Enzymes: Enzymes are responsible for thousands of metabolic processes that sustain life, among them the digestion of food and the synthesis of DNA. (Chapter 4)

Excitotoxin: A class of chemicals that overstimulate neuron receptors in the brain. These neuron receptors allow brain cells to communicate with each other, but when exposed to excitotoxins they fire impulses so quickly they become exhausted. They bind to a nerve cell receptor, stimulate the cell ultimately damaging or causing its death. (Excitotoxic) damage. Common excitotoxins are MSG and aspartame. (Appendix D)

Fat: A major source of energy in the diet and is one of the three main macro nutrients: **fat, carbohydrate,** and **protein.** Fats play a vital role in maintaining healthy skin and hair, and promoting healthy cell function. (Chapter 4)

Free radical: An especially reactive atom or group of atoms that has one or more unpaired electrons; *Free radicals are* produced in the body by natural biological processes or introduced from an outside source (as tobacco smoke, toxins, or pollutants) and can damage cells, proteins, and DNA by altering their chemical structure. They are an unavoidable by-product of daily living. They can harm the fats in our cells with the damage from free radicals leading to age related diseases. Antioxidants from fruits and vegetables keep the damage in check. (Chapter 2)

Ghee: Clarified butter with many health benefits made from organic sweet cream. (Chapter 1)

Gluten: The lectin(protein) in wheat, barley and rye which binds to the intestine. (Chapter 1)

GMO's: Genetically modified foods (or GM foods) are foods produced from organisms that have had specific changes introduced into their DNA using the methods of genetic engineering (Appendix D)

Hemp seeds: They contain all the essential amino acids and essential fatty acids necessary to maintain healthy human life. These fatty acids are in a perfect ratio to meet human nutritional needs.(Chapter 1)

HGH: The naturally occurring growth hormone released by the human pituitary gland. Human growth hormone release in the body slows with aging. (Chapter 2)

Himalayan salt: Himalayan salt mined deep inside the Himalayan mountains containing a high mineral content. The darker the color the more minerals in the salt. (Chapter 4)

Homeostasis: A process that maintains the stability of the human body's internal environment in response to external changes. (Chapter 2)

Inflammation: Is the body's attempt at self-protection to remove harmful stimuli and begin the healing process and is also a part of the body's immune response. Smoking, stress, alcohol and overeating are some causes of inflammation. (Chapter 1)

Leaky Gut Syndrome: A condition where the intestinal wall has become permeable due to undigested food particles, toxins, and microbes that have weakened the cells in the GI tract. The immune system sensing these invaders as foreign, launches an attack as they enter the bloodstream.

Lectin: Proteins in foods, chiefly of plant origin, which bind specifically to certain sugars and cause agglutination of particular cell types. (Chapter 1)

Leptin: The hormone in the brain which tells us when we are full. (Appendix D)

Naturopathy: A system or method of treating disease that employs no surgery or synthetic drugs but uses special diets, herbs, vitamins, massage, etc., to assist the natural healing processes. (Chapter 1)

Obesogens: Chemicals that have been found to disrupt the endocrine system and promote weight gain and obesity. (Appendix D)

Omentum: This is a layer of fat underneath the muscles in the stomach. It's an energy source for the organs and travels to the liver and is shipped to arteries where it is linked to cholesterol problems. Loosing weight reduces this harmful fat. (Appendix D)

Protein: One of the three nutrients used as energy sources (calories) by the body. Proteins are essential components of the muscle, skin, and bones. Proteins are found in all plant and animal sources in varying amounts. (Chapter 1)

Raw unrefined coconut oil: A non-hydrogenated cholesterol free oil which kills harmful pathogens. With antimicrobial, anti-fungal and anti bacterial properties coconut oil is one of the healthiest oils containing medium-chain fatty acids easily converted to energy. (Appendix D)

Xenoestrogens: Imitate estrogen. They can be either synthetic or natural chemical compounds. Synthetic xenoestrogens are widely used industrial compounds, such as PCBs, BPA and phthalates. Natural xenoestrogens include phytoestrogens which are plant-derived xenoestrogens. Because the primary route of exposure to these compounds is by consumption of these plants, they are sometimes called "dietary estrogens". (Appendix D)

HIS FOODS

Thank you for reading my book. I hope it will provide you with information to improve your well being.

Norma Jean

I can be contacted at

www.normajeanpublications.wordpress.com

Or by e-mail

normajeanpub@gmx.com

REFERENCES

References

HEALTH AND NUTRITION SECRETS that can save your life, Russell L. Blaylock, M.D.
> Albuquerque, NM. Health Press.

EXCITOTOXINS, The Taste that Kills, Russell L. Blaylock, M.D. 1997 Albuquerque, NM.
> Health Press NA Inc.

EAT RIGHT 4 YOUR TYPE, Dr. Peter J. D' Adamo with Catherine Whitney, 1996 G.P. Putnam's
> SONS

FREE RADICALS: A MAJOR CAUSE OF AGING AND DISEASE, Consumer Health
> Organization March 1995 volume 18 issue 2

ALZHEIMER'S ASSOCIATION ALZHEIMER'S DISEASE FACTS AND FIGURES, alz.org

INTERNAL CLEANSING is an OLD MOVEMENT, Lee DuBelle 1998 Tempe, Arizona

PROPER FOOD COMBINING WORKS LIVING TESTIMONY, Lee DuBelle, Tempe, Arizona

ARE BIO TECH FOODS SAFE TO EAT? Web MD article from Food Safety

THE BLUE ZONES, Dan Buettner, 2010 National Geographic

FREEDOM FROM DISEASE, Hari Sharma, M.D. 1993 Veda Pub.

THE COCONUT OIL MIRACLE, BRUCE FIFE,C.N. N.D 2004 PICADILLY BOOKS

HIS FOODS